FIBROMYALGIA DIET

COOKBOOK

Nutrient-Rich, Anti-Inflammatory Recipes To Manage Pain, Boost Energy, And Improve Quality Of Life

DR ELIAN GRIFFIN

DISCLAIMER

The nutritional recommendations and recipes in this book are meant solely for informative reasons. They are not meant to replace the counsel, diagnosis, or care of a qualified medical expert. If you have any doubts about a medical condition or dietary requirements, you should always see your physician or another trained healthcare expert.

All reasonable efforts have been taken by the author and publisher to ensure that the information contained in this book is correct as of the date of publication. Recommendations may alter, though, as medical knowledge is always changing. When using any of the recipes or instructions found here, the user assumes all liability and assumes no risk, whether personal or otherwise. People who have certain dietary requirements or medical issues should speak with a healthcare provider for personalized guidance. The given recipes are only ideas; you may need to adjust them to suit your own nutritional needs, tastes, and tolerances.

When you use this book, you agree to release the publisher, the author, and their representatives from any liability for any claims, damages, liabilities, costs, or expenditures resulting from your use of the book.

TABLE OF CONTENTS

ABOUT THE BOOK

The "Fibromyalgia Diet Cookbook" is an invaluable resource for anyone attempting to manage the symptoms of fibromyalgia through dietary interventions. Given the significant influence that diet has on health, particularly for those who have fibromyalgia, the cookbook highlights the critical role that a well-balanced, nutrient-rich diet plays in reducing symptoms and improving overall health.

Debunking common misconceptions surrounding fibromyalgia, highlighting the personalized nature of dietary approaches, and providing readers with valuable resources for deeper understanding, this book provides readers with a comprehensive foundation to better understand the complex nature of fibromyalgia and how dietary adjustments can mitigate discomfort and improve daily life.

The centerpiece of the cookbook is its emphasis on nutritional foundations designed especially for individuals with fibromyalgia.

It provides readers with the tools to create meals that support optimal health and symptom management by defining key nutrients and dietary guidelines. It also emphasizes hydration and offers advice on how to improve nutrient absorption, which further amplifies the impact of dietary modifications.

Beyond theory, the cookbook provides helpful advice on how to choose foods that support symptom relief. It offers a range of anti-inflammatory options, nutrient-dense foods, and easy-to-digest options catered to sensitive stomachs. Sample meal plans and recipes serve as both inspiration and practical tools for quick implementation, making it easy for readers to incorporate these dietary changes into their everyday lives.

Techniques for customized meal planning and preparation are just as important as strategies to steer clear of trigger foods and allergens that are known to worsen symptoms. Useful advice on healthy cooking practices and meal prep reduces fatigue and optimizes nutritional value, enabling readers to sustainably manage their energy levels and general well-being.

In addition, the cookbook discusses the integrative approach to managing fibromyalgia, which incorporates stress management and mindful eating practices in addition to dietary adjustments. It also recognizes the social and lifestyle aspects of coping with dietary modifications, providing advice on how to handle social situations, and getting support from family and friends.

The cookbook uses technology to plan meals and track progress, making it easier to achieve and maintain wellness.

Finally, the inclusion of extensive resources guarantees that readers will have support throughout their journey toward better health. These resources range from online communities and additional reading materials to healthcare professionals with experience in dietary management.

CHAPTER ONE

FIBROMYALGIA DIET INTRODUCTION

DESCRIBE HOW DIET AFFECTS FIBROMYALGIA SYMPTOMS

To effectively manage fibromyalgia, it is important to understand how diet affects symptoms. A lot of people who have fibromyalgia find that certain foods either help or worsen their symptoms. For example, foods high in sugar, processed ingredients, or caffeine may cause increased levels of pain or fatigue. Conversely, a diet high in anti-inflammatory foods, such as fruits, vegetables, lean proteins, and healthy fats, may help to reduce symptoms like pain sensitivity and fatigue.

Studies indicate that inflammation may be a major factor in fibromyalgia and that the body can be affected by certain dietary choices that either increase or decrease inflammation. Therefore, the Fibromyalgia Diet Cookbook's dietary recommendations and recipes are based on the understanding that a diet that promotes overall health and reduces inflammation may lead to improved quality of life and better symptom management for fibromyalgia sufferers.

THE VALUE OF A NUTRIENT-RICH, BALANCED DIET

For those who are managing fibromyalgia, a balanced and nutrient-rich diet is especially important. A healthy diet promotes overall immune function, energy levels, and mood stabilization, all of which can have a direct impact on fibromyalgia symptoms. For example, deficiencies in specific vitamins and minerals, like vitamin D, magnesium, and B vitamins, have been associated with increased pain and fatigue in fibromyalgia patients. As such, making sure you are getting enough of these nutrients through diet becomes imperative.

A balanced diet also helps to keep blood sugar levels stable, which can help people with fibromyalgia avoid the energy crashes and mood swings that they frequently experience. People can support their body's natural healing processes and possibly lessen the severity of their symptoms by focusing on whole foods that contain a variety of nutrients. The Fibromyalgia Diet Cookbook highlights the value of balanced nutrition by providing recipes that are not only delicious but also created to provide essential nutrients needed for optimal health and symptom management.

ADVANTAGES OF CHANGING YOUR DIET IN CERTAIN WAYS

Beyond just relieving symptoms, implementing specialized dietary modifications for fibromyalgia can yield many advantages.

These modifications typically involve cutting back on or avoiding processed foods, sugars, and artificial additives—all of which are known to exacerbate inflammation and worsen symptoms—in favor of increasing the intake of whole foods, such as fresh produce, whole grains, lean meats, and fresh fruits and vegetables, which can supply vital nutrients and anti-inflammatory compounds that promote general health.

A fibromyalgia diet can help people feel less pain, sleep better, think clearer, and have more energy. These benefits can greatly improve everyday functioning and overall quality of life. The Fibromyalgia Diet Cookbook explains these benefits in easy-to-understand terms and offers helpful advice on making long-lasting dietary adjustments that fit personal preferences and health objectives.

AN OVERVIEW OF THE APPROACH AND STRUCTURE OF THE COOKBOOK

To meet the needs of people who are managing fibromyalgia, the Fibromyalgia Diet Cookbook is organized in a way that is both practical and user-friendly. It starts with an introduction that explains the reasoning behind dietary recommendations and offers insights into how specific foods can impact symptoms. The cookbook is then divided into sections that cover different meal types, such as breakfast, lunch, dinner, snacks, and desserts, to provide a thorough approach to daily eating habits.

In addition to providing tips on meal planning, grocery shopping, and modifying recipes to suit specific dietary preferences or restrictions, each recipe in the cookbook is thoughtfully designed to be nourishing, tasty, and simple to make. The cookbook's structured approach to meal preparation and dietary management aims to provide readers with the tools they need to take charge of their nutrition and enhance their general well-being.

HOW TO MAKE THE MOST OF THIS COOKBOOK

To get the most out of the Fibromyalgia Diet Cookbook, you should approach it strategically. Read through the introductory sections to become familiar with the basic ideas behind the diet and how it can help manage fibromyalgia. Then, spend some time looking through the table of contents and recipe index to gain an idea of the wide range of recipes that are offered.

Use the meal planning advice in the cookbook to create well-balanced, gratifying menus that feature a range of flavors and ingredients. Make sure to pay attention to any special instructions or dietary modifications included with each recipe to ensure that it meets your unique needs. Plan your meals based on your personal preferences and nutritional requirements.

Keep a record of your favorite recipes and meal combinations to make meal planning easier in the future. Follow the recipes step-by-step as you start cooking, making sure you have all the necessary ingredients and utensils ready. Don't be afraid to experiment with different recipes and variations to find what works best for you.

You can use nutrition to better control your symptoms and enhance your overall quality of life by following the guidelines in the Fibromyalgia Diet Cookbook.

CHAPTER TWO

KNOWING ABOUT FIBROMYALGIA

SIGNS AND EVALUATION OF FIBROMYALGIA

The first step in comprehending fibromyalgia is identifying its variety of symptoms, which frequently include fatigue, widespread pain, and cognitive difficulties known as "fibro fog." People who have fibromyalgia may also experience increased pain sensitivity, irregular sleep patterns, and mood disturbances like depression or anxiety. Diagnosis can be difficult because symptoms can overlap with other conditions, necessitating a thorough evaluation by a healthcare professional. This evaluation usually entails a thorough medical history, a physical examination to identify tender points, and the exclusion of other potential causes through blood tests and imaging studies.

The journey to effectively managing fibromyalgia begins with awareness of these symptoms and a proactive approach to diagnosis and treatment. Because fibromyalgia symptoms can vary from person to person in intensity and impact, it is important to recognize and document symptom patterns. Individuals can then work with healthcare professionals to develop personalized treatment plans that may include medication, physical therapy, and lifestyle modifications.

THE DIET'S FUNCTION IN SYMPTOM MANAGEMENT

While there is no one "fibromyalgia diet," certain dietary approaches can help alleviate symptoms and improve quality of life. For example, maintaining a balanced diet rich in fruits, vegetables, lean proteins, and whole grains can provide essential nutrients and support energy levels.

Avoiding or moderating intake of caffeine, alcohol, and processed foods may also help reduce symptoms like fatigue and digestive issues. Diet plays a crucial role in managing symptoms of fibromyalgia by supporting overall health and addressing specific symptom triggers.

Furthermore, some people find relief by determining and removing potential allergens or food sensitivities by following an elimination diet, which entails methodically removing suspected trigger foods from the diet and reintroducing them one at a time to watch for any negative reactions. Keeping a food diary can help with tracking symptoms and identifying patterns associated with dietary decisions. People can customize their diet to meet their unique needs and effectively manage fibromyalgia symptoms by working closely with a registered dietitian or healthcare provider.

FREQUENTLY HELD MYTHS REGARDING FIBROMYALGIA

Some common misconceptions about fibromyalgia include the idea that it is only a psychological disorder or that it is not a real medical condition; in fact, fibromyalgia is a complex disorder that affects the nervous system and can cause widespread pain and other debilitating symptoms. Another common misconception is that all fibromyalgia sufferers have the same symptoms, even though symptoms can vary greatly amongst individuals.

While there is currently no cure for fibromyalgia, a multimodal treatment approach that includes medications, lifestyle modifications, and complementary therapies can help improve quality of life. Education and awareness about the realities of fibromyalgia are crucial in dispelling these myths and promoting understanding and support for those living with the condition. Another common misconception is that fibromyalgia is incurable or that the only option for managing symptoms is to take medication.

PERSONALIZED DIETARY APPROACHES' SIGNIFICANCE

What works for one person may not work for another, underscoring the significance of customizing dietary recommendations to specific symptoms and health goals. Personalized approaches may involve identifying and avoiding trigger foods that exacerbate symptoms such as inflammation or digestive issues. They may also involve optimizing nutrient intake to support overall health and energy levels. Personalized dietary approaches are crucial for managing fibromyalgia because they acknowledge the unique triggers and sensitivities of each individual.

Personalized dietary approaches can also encourage people to take charge of their health and well-being. Through trial and error with various foods and tracking how they affect symptoms, people can learn how their diet affects their fibromyalgia symptoms. Working with a registered dietitian or healthcare provider can help individuals create a personalized nutrition plan that suits their needs and preferences. In the end, personalized dietary approaches provide a proactive and empowering way to manage fibromyalgia.

SOURCES FOR ADDITIONAL KNOWLEDGE

If you would like more information about fibromyalgia and how it can be managed with diet, several resources can be helpful. Trusted websites run by national health organizations or respectable medical centers frequently have extensive guides and articles about the symptoms, diagnosis, and available treatments of fibromyalgia. Books written by medical professionals who specialize in fibromyalgia or nutrition can offer in-depth analyses and helpful guidance on dietary strategies.

Individuals can also benefit from the social support that support groups and online communities devoted to fibromyalgia provide by connecting with others who are going through similar struggles. These communities can also offer emotional support, useful advice, and personal experiences regarding managing fibromyalgia symptoms through dietary and lifestyle modifications. Lastly, seeking advice from healthcare professionals such as rheumatologists, pain specialists, and registered dietitians can also provide individualized guidance based on the needs and preferences of each patient.

CHAPTER THREE

CRUCIAL ELEMENTS FOR PEOPLE WITH FIBROMYALGIA

To effectively manage the symptoms of fibromyalgia, it is imperative to ensure that an adequate intake of essential nutrients is maintained. Some of these nutrients are omega-3 fatty acids, which have anti-inflammatory properties and can help reduce pain and stiffness. You can find these in fatty fish like salmon, flaxseeds, and walnuts. Magnesium is another important nutrient that is known to help relax muscles and reduce pain. You can get it in spinach, almonds, and whole grains.

Furthermore, adequate levels of B vitamins, particularly B12 and folate, support nerve function and energy production, which is crucial for managing fatigue and cognitive symptoms associated with fibromyalgia. Antioxidants like vitamins C and E can combat oxidative stress and inflammation; they are abundant in fruits, vegetables, and nuts. Finally, vitamin D plays a significant role in immune function and bone health, which are often compromised in patients with fibromyalgia. Sunlight exposure and fortified foods, such as fortified milk and cereals, are primary sources of vitamin D.

DIETARY RECOMMENDATIONS AND GUIDELINES

Following certain dietary recommendations can have a big impact on how fibromyalgia symptoms are managed. To start, eating an anti-inflammatory diet full of fruits, vegetables, whole grains, and lean proteins can help reduce pain and inflammation. Processed foods, which are high in sugar and unhealthy fats, can also help prevent symptoms from getting worse.

Incorporating small, frequent meals can help prevent energy crashes and maintain consistent nutrient intake throughout the day; for those who are sensitive to certain foods, keeping a food diary to identify triggers like gluten, dairy, or artificial additives can aid in symptom management.

Maintaining regular meal timings is also essential to stabilize blood sugar levels, which can affect mood and energy levels.

Hydration is key; drinking enough water supports healthy muscle function, mental clarity, and general well-being. Incorporating herbal teas and infused water into meals can add interest and maintain proper hydration levels. Lastly, speaking with a medical professional or registered dietitian can offer individualized dietary advice based on symptoms and individual needs.

CREATING A PLATE THAT'S BALANCED AND FIBROMYALGIA-FRIENDLY

Meal plans for managing fibromyalgia should balance macronutrients and include nutrient-dense foods. Complex carbohydrates, such as whole grains, offer sustained energy and fiber to support digestive health. Carbohydrates should be paired with lean proteins, such as turkey, chicken, tofu, or legumes, to support satiety and muscle repair.

Include a range of vibrant vegetables to guarantee a spectrum of vitamins, minerals, and antioxidants. Magnesium is abundant in leafy greens like spinach and kale, while colorful veggies like bell peppers and tomatoes offer vitamin C. Heart-healthy fats from avocados, olive oil, and nuts help reduce inflammation and support heart health.

A balanced and enjoyable diet that supports overall health and symptom management should emphasize moderation in portion sizes to avoid overeating, which can lead to discomfort and fatigue. Experiment with herbs and spices for flavor instead of excessive salt or sugar. Include omega-3 fatty acids through fatty fish like salmon or plant-based sources like chia seeds and flaxseeds to combat inflammation and support brain function.

THE VALUE OF HYDRATION AND HOW IT AFFECTS SYMPTOMS

Water is necessary for maintaining muscle tone and joint lubrication, which helps to reduce stiffness and discomfort. Adequate hydration also supports kidney function, which helps to eliminate toxins that can exacerbate symptoms. All of these benefits contribute to the management of fibromyalgia symptoms. Hydration also supports cellular function, digestion, and cognitive clarity.

Herbal teas and infused waters offer flavor without added sugars or caffeine, promoting hydration throughout the day. Avoiding excessive caffeine and alcohol intake, which can dehydrate the body and disrupt sleep patterns, is crucial for symptom management. Fruits and vegetables with high water content, like cucumbers, melons, and citrus fruits, add variety and additional hydration benefits.

Urine color can be used as an easy way to check your level of hydration; light yellow means you're well hydrated, and darker colors can mean you're dehydrated. It's best to drink eight glasses or more of water a day, depending on your needs and level of activity.

People with fibromyalgia can improve their overall health and relieve some common symptoms by emphasizing their water intake.

For those with fibromyalgia, maximizing the benefits of dietary choices requires optimizing nutrient absorption: eating foods high in vitamin C, like berries, citrus fruits, and bell peppers, improves iron absorption from plant-based sources like spinach and lentils; eating foods high in probiotics, like kefir, yogurt, and fermented vegetables, supports gut health and improves digestion, which in turn helps absorb nutrients.

Eating in an environment that is conducive to proper digestion and nutrient assimilation is encouraged by chewing food thoroughly and avoiding excessive caffeine and alcohol consumption, which can hinder nutrient absorption and deplete vital vitamins and minerals. Cooking food gently or steaming it retains more nutrients than boiling or frying it, which is beneficial for maintaining vital vitamins and minerals.

Incorporating a range of foods guarantees a diverse nutrient intake, supporting overall health and symptom management in fibromyalgia sufferers. Additionally, supplementing with digestive enzymes or probiotics under a doctor's supervision can help with nutrient breakdown and absorption, especially for those with digestive problems or food sensitivities.

CHAPTER FOUR

FOODS TO AVOID

FOODS THAT CAN AGGRAVATE SYMPTOMS AND CAUSE TRIGGERS

To effectively manage the symptoms of fibromyalgia, it is important to identify the foods that exacerbate pain, fatigue, and overall discomfort. Common trigger foods include processed foods high in artificial additives and refined sugars, which can lead to inflammation and exacerbate symptoms.

Caffeine and alcohol can also disrupt sleep patterns and increase sensitivity to pain in fibromyalgia sufferers. Dairy products and gluten-containing grains can also cause digestive problems and joint pain in certain individuals.

Keep a food journal and record any symptoms you experience after eating particular foods. Elimination diets, in which you temporarily cut out suspected trigger foods from your diet and then add them back one at a time, can be very helpful in determining which foods exacerbate your symptoms. Whole, unprocessed foods, like fruits, vegetables, lean proteins, and whole grains, are high in nutrients and do not contain the additives and preservatives found in processed foods.

COMMON SENSITIVITIES AND ALLERGENS

Allergies and food sensitivities are common in fibromyalgia sufferers; common allergens include nuts, shellfish, eggs, and soy products. Allergies can cause allergic reactions, and worsen pre-existing symptoms like inflammation and digestive problems, or both. Food sensitivities, on the other hand, sometimes cause delayed symptoms like headaches, joint pain, and bloating.

Identifying allergens and sensitivities can be accomplished through allergy testing or working with a healthcare provider who specializes in dietary management. Removing possible allergens from your diet and reintroducing them gradually can help determine which foods may be problematic.

If you suspect allergies or sensitivities, choose allergen-free options like gluten-free grains or nut-free milk. This strategy lets you enjoy a varied diet while reducing discomfort and effectively managing symptoms of fibromyalgia.

SYNTHETIC ADDITIVES AND THEIR EFFECTS

Preservatives, flavor enhancers, and artificial sweeteners are examples of artificial additives that can exacerbate fibromyalgia symptoms. These additives are frequently found in processed foods, snacks, and beverages. They may cause inflammation, digestive problems, and general exhaustion. Aspartame is one type of artificial sweetener that has been linked to increased pain sensitivity in fibromyalgia sufferers.

You can prevent artificial additives by carefully reading food labels, cooking from scratch gives you control over ingredients and helps you avoid additives that worsen symptoms, and focusing on fresh produce, lean proteins, and whole grains will nourish your body without the harmful effects of artificial additives.

When choosing sweeteners, go for natural ones like honey or maple syrup.

A registered dietitian or other healthcare professional knowledgeable about fibromyalgia can offer guidance and support in identifying personal triggers. Each person with fibromyalgia may have different trigger foods and sensitivities, so personalized strategies for identifying these triggers may include keeping a detailed food diary, tracking symptoms, and noting any patterns or reactions after meals.

Reintroducing suspected trigger foods one at a time after gradually removing them from your diet can help pinpoint specific triggers.

Track your daily food intake and symptoms using apps or journals. This will help you make connections between specific foods and flare-ups of symptoms. Be methodical and patient when identifying triggers; patterns may take some time to notice.

Once triggers are identified, concentrate on creating a personalized meal plan that steers clear of trigger foods while providing enough nutrition and enjoyment from food choices.

SUBSTITUTES FOR OFTEN TROUBLESOME FOODS

Experimenting with different cooking methods and recipes can help you find enjoyable alternatives that support your health and well-being. For example, you can replace dairy products with plant-based alternatives like almond milk or coconut yogurt; for people who are sensitive to nightshade vegetables like tomatoes and peppers, try non-nightshade alternatives like squash and sweet potatoes; and for those who are sensitive to other common problematic foods, try substituting gluten-containing grains with gluten-free options like quinoa, brown rice, or oats.

A balanced approach to nutrition and customized dietary adjustments can help you optimize your diet to support your health goals and improve your quality of life with fibromyalgia.

Choosing whole, nutrient-dense foods ensures you receive essential vitamins and minerals without aggravating symptoms. Include a variety of fruits, vegetables, lean proteins, and healthy fats in your diet to maintain overall health and manage fibromyalgia symptoms effectively. Be aware of food labels and ingredients to avoid artificial additives and preservatives that can exacerbate symptoms.

CHAPTER FIVE

MEAL PLANNING AND PREPARATION

A COMPREHENSIVE GUIDE TO MEAL PLANNING

To effectively manage a diet for fibromyalgia, you must first set aside time each week to plan your meals. To start, make a list of foods that are good for fibromyalgia, such as fruits, vegetables, whole grains, and lean proteins.

You should also consider your dietary preferences and any foods that make your symptoms worse. To maintain consistent energy levels, plan balanced meals that include protein, healthy fats, and complex carbohydrates.

Next, make a weekly meal plan that includes breakfast, lunch, dinner, and snacks. Then, choose recipes that are easy to make and emphasize reducing prep time and stress. You can also batch-cook some dishes to save time on busy days. Finally, use containers to store prepared meals in the refrigerator or freezer so that they are always available. Aim for variety to ensure that you get a range of nutrients.

Last but not least, make periodic reviews of your plan and tweak it according to your energy and mood. Stock your kitchen with basic ingredients like herbs, spices, and pantry items to add flavor without using processed foods. Eating a healthy and well-balanced diet can be achieved by adhering to a structured meal plan.

TIPS FOR PREPARING MEALS AND BATCH COOKING

When it comes to managing a fibromyalgia diet, batch cooking is invaluable. Pick a day when you have more energy, like the weekend, and make larger batches of meals. Go for recipes that freeze well and reheat easily, like soups, stews, and casseroles. For hands-off, minimally labor-intensive cooking, use a slow cooker or instant pot.

To ensure you always have wholesome options on hand, even during flare-ups, invest in high-quality, freezer- and microwave-safe storage containers to store your batch-cooked meals. Label containers with dates and contents for simple identification. Portion meals into individual servings to grab and go as needed.

One way to simplify meal times and support your fibromyalgia management is to incorporate batch cooking and meal prep into your routine. Some ideas for meal prep include pre-cooking grains like brown rice or quinoa, making smoothie packs with frozen fruits and greens, and washing and chopping vegetables ahead of time.

EASY AND QUICK RECIPES FOR A BUSY DAY

Smoothies or overnight oats for breakfast can be made ahead of time and customized with nutrient-dense add-ins like chia seeds or protein powder.

For lunch, salads with pre-cooked proteins like canned tuna or grilled chicken offer a balanced meal with little work. These kinds of recipes are great for busy days when dealing with fibromyalgia.

Dinner recipes might be stir-fries with frozen or fresh veggies and lean protein, or sheet pan meals where everything cooks at once for minimal cleanup. Seasonings and herbs can boost flavor without adding extra sodium or calories. Shortcuts like canned beans or pre-cut vegetables can shorten cooking times.

Keep healthy snacks close at hand to avoid reaching for processed foods. You can maintain a nutritious diet without sacrificing taste or convenience by including quick and easy recipes in your meal plan. Snack options can include yogurt with fresh fruit, nuts, or hummus with vegetable sticks for a quick energy boost.

MODIFYING RECIPES TO MEET VARIOUS DIETARY REQUIREMENTS

When managing fibromyalgia, it's critical to modify recipes to accommodate varying dietary needs. To begin, identify your dietary preferences or restrictions, such as low FODMAP, dairy-free, or gluten-free, and search for substitute ingredients that satisfy your requirements without sacrificing flavor or nutritional value.

Use plant-based milk alternatives like almond milk or coconut milk in recipes; experiment with dairy-free cheeses or nutritional yeast for added flavor; for gluten-free diets, replace wheat flour with almond flour or gluten-free oats in baking recipes; and use tamari instead of soy sauce to avoid gluten-containing ingredients.

Reduced fermentable carbohydrates, which can worsen digestive symptoms, are the main focus of low-FODMAPS diets. Low-FODMAPS ingredients include leafy greens, carrots, and proteins like chicken or tofu. Garlic-infused oil can be used in place of cloves of garlic, and servings of high-FODMAPS foods, such as onions and garlic, should be limited.

You can enjoy tasty, satisfying meals that assist your fibromyalgia management by modifying recipes to suit your nutritional needs; try different ingredients and cooking methods to see what works best for you.

ESSENTIALS FOR A FIBROMYALGIA DIET: A SHOPPING LIST

A fibromyalgia diet shopping list guarantees you have the supplies you need for wholesome meals. To start, add lean proteins like turkey, chicken, fish, or tofu. These provide the essential amino acids needed for muscle growth and repair. Then, add high-fiber foods like quinoa, brown rice, and oats to help maintain a healthy digestive system and stabilize blood sugar levels.

Choose heart-healthy fats like avocados, olive oil, and nuts to improve nutrient absorption. Include a variety of fruits and vegetables rich in antioxidants and vitamins, such as berries, leafy greens, bell peppers, and sweet potatoes. These foods help reduce inflammation and support overall immune function.

For flavor enhancement without added sugars or salts, stock up on pantry staples like herbs, spices, and low-sodium broths. For complex carbohydrates that give you long-lasting energy, choose whole grains like buckwheat noodles or whole-wheat pasta. Depending on your dietary needs, think about dairy or dairy substitutes like almond milk or yogurt.

You can make balanced meals that support your overall health and well-being by organizing your shopping list around fibromyalgia-friendly foods. You can also make sure you always have the products you need on hand by reviewing and updating your list regularly based on your preferences and meal plan.

RECIPES FOR BREAKFAST

When creating breakfast recipes for a fibromyalgia diet, it's important to concentrate on foods that are high in nutrients and simple to digest. For example, a spinach and feta omelet, which combines the protein from eggs with the vitamins and minerals in spinach and the richness of feta cheese, supports muscle function and provides essential nutrients for general health. Another excellent option is a smoothie bowl with berries, nuts, and seeds; this breakfast is simple to make and can be customized with ingredients like chia seeds or almond milk for extra flavor and nutrition. Refined sugars and processed grains should be avoided as they can aggravate fibromyalgia symptoms.

Lunch should be about well-balanced, nutrient-dense meals that keep you going all day. A great option is a salad of quinoa and vegetables with a lemon-tahini dressing. Quinoa is a gluten-free grain that is high in protein and fiber, and the vegetables offer vitamins and minerals that are important for immune system health and general well-being. The lemon-tahini dressing gives the salad a creamy texture and healthy fats, which makes it a nutritious and satisfying dish. Another great option is a turkey and avocado wrap made with gluten-free tortillas. The turkey is a lean protein that supports muscle health, and the avocado is a source of fiber and healthy fats. This meal is easy to put together and can be topped with extra veggies like lettuce, tomatoes, and cucumbers for flavor and nutrition.

When planning dinner for a fibromyalgia diet, aim for meals that are comforting yet nutritious, supporting overall health and well-being. One delicious option is a salmon and quinoa bowl with roasted vegetables. Salmon is rich in omega-3 fatty acids, which have anti-inflammatory properties and support brain health. Quinoa provides protein and fiber, while roasted vegetables like sweet potatoes and broccoli add vitamins, minerals, and fiber. This bowl is easy to prepare and can be seasoned with herbs and spices for added flavor without relying on salt. Another great choice is a vegetable stir-fry with tofu or lean chicken breast. Stir-fries are versatile and can include a variety of colorful vegetables like bell peppers, carrots, and snap peas, providing antioxidants and fiber. Tofu or chicken adds protein, making this dish both satisfying and nutritious. It's essential to avoid heavy sauces and excessive salt, which can contribute to inflammation and discomfort for those with fibromyalgia.

Breakfast, lunch, and dinner ideas that support a fibromyalgia diet by emphasizing nutrient-dense ingredients that support overall health and well-being. These recipes can help manage symptoms and improve energy levels throughout the day by incorporating lean proteins, healthy fats, and plenty of fruits and vegetables. Each dish is simple to make and can be tailored to suit individual dietary preferences and tastes while avoiding ingredients that may exacerbate fibromyalgia symptoms. Meal planning can play a big role in managing fibromyalgia and promoting overall wellness.

CHAPTER SIX

COOKING METHODS AND ADVICE

OPTIMAL COOKING TECHNIQUES FOR PRESERVING NUTRIENTS

Choosing the right cooking techniques can make a big difference in nutrient retention and overall health benefits when preparing meals for a fibromyalgia diet. Techniques like steaming, baking, and poaching preserve vital vitamins and minerals that might be lost during high-heat cooking. For example, steaming vegetables preserve their crisp texture and vibrant color while preserving water-soluble vitamins like vitamin C and B vitamins. Baking or roasting lean proteins like chicken or fish guarantees they stay juicy and tender without adding extra fats, which is good for controlling weight and inflammation that is frequently linked to fibromyalgia.

Slow cooking or using a crockpot is also a great way to prepare fibromyalgia-friendly meals because it allows ingredients to simmer gently over low heat, enhancing flavors and tenderness without the need for excessive stirring or monitoring. These methods not only preserve nutrients but also make meal preparation easier and more enjoyable for people managing fibromyalgia symptoms.

Sautéing with minimal oil or using heart-healthy oils like olive or avocado oil, which are rich in monounsaturated fats and can support cardiovascular health, is another healthy cooking technique.

METHODS FOR ENHANCING FLAVOR WITHOUT ADDING ADDITIVES

It is possible to improve the flavor of fibromyalgia diet recipes without using additives or too much salt, which can worsen symptoms. Adding fresh herbs and spices, like turmeric, ginger, basil, and cilantro, not only gives richness and complexity to meals but also has anti-inflammatory qualities that can help reduce fibromyalgia pain, and also brightens flavors without adding sodium.

Both balsamic and apple cider vinegar can add tanginess and balance to dishes without requiring heavy sauces or dressings.

Further enhancing flavors can be achieved by experimenting with different cooking techniques, such as marinating proteins in herbs and citrus before cooking, or by using aromatic vegetables like onions and garlic as a base for soups and stews. By concentrating on enhancing flavors through wholesome ingredients, people can create satisfying meals that support overall well-being and effectively manage symptoms. Natural umami-rich ingredients like mushrooms, tomatoes, and soy sauce alternatives like coconut aminos are examples of ingredients that do this.

ADVICE FOR LOWERING FATIGUE ASSOCIATED WITH COOKING

The key to managing fibromyalgia is energy conservation during daily activities, which includes meal preparation. To reduce fatigue associated with cooking, meal planning, and batch cooking are very beneficial. This involves making larger quantities of fibromyalgia-friendly recipes and putting them in individual servings for convenient reheating during the week. Slow cookers, food processors, and ergonomic utensils are some of the kitchen tools and gadgets that can simplify meal preparation and lessen physical strain.

Keeping frequently used ingredients and tools readily available in the kitchen can also help you save time and energy. For instance, you can make cooking easier by keeping spices and herbs close at hand or storing pantry items in stackable containers.

You can also avoid burnout by breaking down cooking tasks into smaller, more manageable steps and taking breaks when necessary. You can also prevent cooking burnout by scheduling rest periods in between cooking tasks, asking family members for assistance, or ordering takeout on particularly difficult days.

APPLIANCES AND KITCHEN TOOLS FOR SIMPLIFIED MEAL PREPARATION

Having the right kitchen tools and appliances can help people with fibromyalgia prepare meals more effectively and enjoyably. Get good quality knives with ergonomic handles to prevent wrist strain and guarantee accurate ingredient cutting. Food processors or blenders are great for chopping vegetables, pureeing sauces, and blending smoothies, providing convenience and versatility when making fibromyalgia-friendly meals. A slow cooker or crockpot can make cooking easier by letting ingredients simmer gently for several hours, producing tender and flavorful dishes with little effort on the part of the cook.

Adjustable measuring spoons and cups ensure precise portioning of ingredients without the need for multiple utensils; non-stick cookware can also facilitate cooking and cleaning processes, minimizing the use of oils and fats while preventing ingredients from sticking; people can maximize their cooking experience, conserve energy, and focus on creating nutritious meals that support their health goals by investing in these kitchen essentials. Other helpful gadgets include silicone spatulas and utensils, which are gentle on cookware and easy to clean, reducing the physical strain associated with stirring and mixing.

PUTTING TOGETHER NUTRITIOUS AND DELICIOUS MEALS

Combining nutrient-dense ingredients with inventive cooking methods is the key to creating meals that are both flavorful and balanced for a fibromyalgia diet. To start, include a range of vibrant fruits and vegetables to supply vital vitamins, minerals, and antioxidants. Lean proteins like chicken, turkey, fish, and plant-based sources like beans and lentils support muscle health and energy levels overall. Whole grains like quinoa, brown rice, and oats contribute fiber and complex carbohydrates that promote satiety and stable blood sugar levels.

To keep meals interesting and fulfilling, try experimenting with different cooking techniques and flavor profiles.

For instance, use vegetable or bone broth as a base for hearty soups and stews, then add herbs and spices for additional flavor depth. Make salads with a range of textures and flavors, such as crunchy nuts and seeds, creamy avocado, and tart vinaigrettes made with olive oil and vinegar. Finally, include healthy fats from sources like avocados, nuts, and seeds to support brain health and improve meal satisfaction.

It is possible to prepare meals that satisfy dietary requirements while also being delicious and promoting overall well-being by emphasizing nutrient-rich ingredients and mindful cooking techniques. Trying out new recipes and customizing them to individual tastes and dietary needs guarantees that every meal is satisfying and nourishing, supporting long-term health and fibromyalgia sufferers' ability to manage their symptoms.

CHAPTER SEVEN

TECHNIQUES FOR PRESERVING A HEALTHY WEIGHT

Incorporating a variety of colorful fruits and vegetables, lean proteins, and whole grains into your meals will ensure you're getting essential vitamins and minerals. A balanced approach that takes into account both lifestyle factors and nutrition is necessary to achieve and maintain a healthy weight with fibromyalgia.

Start by focusing on portion control and mindful eating habits. This means paying attention to hunger and fullness cues, choosing nutrient-dense foods, and avoiding processed sugars and unhealthy fats.

Regular physical activity is also important for weight management and improving overall well-being. Choose low-impact exercises like walking, swimming, or yoga that are gentle on joints but still effective in burning calories and building strength. Consistency is key, so aim for at least 30 minutes of exercise most days of the week. Additionally, staying hydrated is crucial for overall health and can help manage the symptoms of fibromyalgia. Drink plenty of water throughout the day and limit sugary beverages.

Another crucial element of managing weight with fibromyalgia is controlling stress levels, which can lead to overeating or unhealthy food choices. You can support your weight management goals by practicing relaxation techniques like deep breathing, meditation, or gentle stretching. Lastly, you can tailor a plan that meets your specific needs and goals by seeking support from healthcare professionals or groups that specialize in fibromyalgia and weight management.

MAINTAINING EQUILIBRIUM ENERGY THROUGHOUT THE DAY

Eating a balanced breakfast that includes protein, healthy fats, and complex carbohydrates to provide sustained energy is a good way to balance your energy levels with fibromyalgia. Other healthy breakfast options include Greek yogurt with berries and nuts or oatmeal with seeds and fruit. Throughout the day, try to eat smaller, more frequent meals and snacks to avoid blood sugar spikes and dips.

Include high-fiber foods like fruits, vegetables, whole grains, and legumes; these can help stabilize blood sugar levels and support sustained energy; steer clear of processed foods and refined sugars, which can cause abrupt swings in energy levels; also, watch how much caffeine you consume—a small amount can give you a quick energy boost, but too much can cause sleep disturbances and exhaustion.

In addition, prioritize adequate rest and sleep hygiene to support overall energy levels. Create a relaxing bedtime routine, stick to a consistent sleep schedule, and make sure your sleep environment is conducive to restful sleep. These strategies combined can help you manage energy levels effectively throughout the day. Keep in mind that dehydration can exacerbate symptoms of fatigue commonly associated with fibromyalgia. Drink water frequently throughout the day.

Start with low-impact exercises like walking, swimming, or cycling, which are gentle on joints but still effective in improving cardiovascular fitness and muscle strength. Gradually increase the duration and intensity of your workouts as tolerated, aiming for at least 150 minutes of moderate aerobic activity per week. Exercise is beneficial for managing fibromyalgia symptoms, including pain, fatigue, and stiffness, as well as supporting weight management and overall health.

Practices such as yoga or tai chi can also help improve balance, coordination, and mindfulness, which may be beneficial for managing stress and enhancing overall well-being. Listen to your body and pace yourself; it's okay to modify exercises or take breaks as needed to avoid exacerbating symptoms. Incorporate flexibility and stretching exercises to improve range of motion and reduce muscle tension.

Maintaining muscle mass and supporting joint stability are important goals of strength training.

Exercises that target major muscle groups, like squats, lunges, and upper body presses, can be performed with light weights or resistance bands. Proper form and technique are key to maximizing benefits and preventing injury. Warming up before exercise and cooling down afterward can help prevent soreness and stiffness in the muscles.

MODIFYING NUTRITION TO ENCOURAGE ENERGY PRODUCTION

Starting with incorporating whole grains, legumes, and vegetables into your meals, which release glucose slowly into the bloodstream to help maintain steady energy levels, is a good place to start for a diet that supports energy production with fibromyalgia. Pairing carbohydrates with lean proteins like chicken, fish, tofu, or beans will help promote satiety and support muscle repair and growth.

Avoid trans fats and limit saturated fats found in processed foods and red meat, as these can contribute to inflammation and worsen symptoms of fibromyalgia;

limit your intake of alcohol and caffeine, which can interfere with sleep and energy levels; and include healthy fats, such as avocados, nuts, seeds, and olive oil, in moderation. These fats are essential for brain function and can help you feel fuller for longer.

Consume foods high in antioxidants, such as leafy greens, berries, and colorful vegetables, to help fight the inflammation and oxidative stress linked to fibromyalgia. Consult a registered dietitian with expertise in managing chronic pain or fibromyalgia to create a customized nutrition plan that meets your needs and goals. You can also make educated dietary decisions by monitoring how different foods affect your energy levels and symptoms by keeping a food diary.

MONITORING DEVELOPMENT AND MAKING MODIFICATIONS

Monitoring your physical activity and eating habits is important for tracking your progress with fibromyalgia. You can use a fitness app or journal to record your daily activities, including the amount of time and intensity you spend exercising as well as any symptoms you experience. This information can be used by you and your healthcare team to determine what's working well and where adjustments may be necessary.

It may take several weeks to notice significant improvements in your ability to maintain a healthy weight, so be patient and give yourself time to track your dietary habits. Pay attention to meal timing, portion sizes, and food choices. Note how different foods make you feel in terms of energy levels, pain levels, and overall well-being. Look for trends or triggers that may exacerbate symptoms.

When evaluating your progress over time, use objective metrics like weight, body measurements, or fitness evaluations. Reward yourself for small successes and accomplishments like better sleep or more endurance during workouts. If you encounter obstacles or setbacks, don't give up; instead, use them as teaching moments to improve your strategy and make the required dietary or exercise modifications.

Tracking your progress and making regular adjustments can help you stay motivated and committed to reaching your goals. Speak with your healthcare provider or a multidisciplinary team specializing in fibromyalgia management to review your progress and address any worries or questions you may have. They can offer guidance on modifying your exercise program or nutrition plan to better meet your individual needs and optimize your overall health and well-being.

CHAPTER EIGHT

STRESS REDUCTION AND INTENTIONAL EATING

THE VALUE OF AWARENESS IN EATING BEHAVIORS

To better understand hunger cues and satiety levels—which are frequently disrupted in fibromyalgia due to altered pain perceptions and medication effects—mindful eating is an important practice for people managing their condition. It involves paying full attention to the sensory experience of eating—tasting, smelling, and savoring each bite. In addition, practicing mindfulness reduces overeating tendencies and supports healthier food choices, all of which are crucial for managing symptoms and maintaining overall well-being.

Developing an awareness of your eating environment and food choices is the first step towards incorporating mindfulness into eating habits. Eat nutrient-dense foods, such as fruits, vegetables, lean proteins, and whole grains that support energy levels and reduce inflammation. Chew slowly, savor flavors, and pause between bites to gauge your level of hunger. This method not only improves digestion but also helps better manage fibromyalgia symptoms by lowering stress responses that can exacerbate pain and fatigue. By adopting mindful eating as a daily habit, people can empower themselves to take control of their health and enhance their quality of life.

To sum up, mindful eating involves more than just what you eat—it also involves how you eat. People with fibromyalgia can manage their symptoms and improve their general well-being by cultivating a mindful approach to meals, which supports healthier food choices, improves digestion, lowers stress levels, and ultimately improves quality of life.

METHODS FOR DIETARY STRESS REDUCTION

For people with fibromyalgia, lowering stress levels through nutrition is crucial because stress can aggravate symptoms like pain, exhaustion, and mood swings. One practical method is to include foods high in omega-3 fatty acids, magnesium, and antioxidants in your diet. Omega-3s, which are found in fatty fish like salmon and flaxseeds, help regulate neurotransmitters that affect mood and stress responses. Magnesium-rich foods, like spinach, whole grains, and nuts, support muscle relaxation and reduce tension. Antioxidants, found in fruits and vegetables, fight oxidative stress linked to chronic pain conditions.

A balanced diet that stabilizes blood sugar levels is another way to lessen the effects of stress responses. Eating complex carbohydrates, such as whole grains and legumes, will give you sustained energy and prevent spikes in cortisol, the stress hormone.

Reducing your intake of processed foods, refined sugars, and excessive caffeine will also help you avoid these foods, which can cause inflammation and upset your hormone balance. By emphasizing nutrient-dense foods and mindful eating practices, people can help their bodies better handle stress and lessen the severity of fibromyalgia symptoms.

To sum up, if you choose to incorporate stress-reduction strategies into your diet, you will be selecting foods that support mental and physical health. People with fibromyalgia can benefit from this by giving priority to foods high in antioxidants, magnesium, omega-3 fatty acids, and stable blood sugar levels. This strategy not only helps to manage symptoms but also fosters resilience and enhances quality of life.

MIND-BODY TECHNIQUES FOR THE MANAGEMENT OF PAIN

Techniques like yoga, tai chi, and qigong emphasize gentle movements, breathing exercises, and meditation, which help alleviate muscle stiffness, improve flexibility, and reduce stress. These practices promote relaxation and enhance the body's natural pain-relieving mechanisms, giving fibromyalgia sufferers a sense of empowerment and control over their symptoms. Mind-body practices are crucial in managing pain associated with fibromyalgia, offering holistic approaches that integrate mental and physical well-being.

By focusing on breath awareness and body scans, people can reduce the perceived intensity of pain and improve their ability to cope with discomfort. Adding these mind-body practices into daily routines builds resilience and supports overall well-being, providing an alternative to traditional pain management strategies. Mindfulness meditation is another useful technique that promotes acceptance of pain without judgment or resistance.

In summary, mind-body techniques such as yoga, tai chi, qigong, and mindfulness meditation promote relaxation, reduce muscle tension, and enhance resilience; by incorporating these practices into daily routines, individuals can experience greater physical comfort, emotional balance, and empowerment in managing their chronic condition. Mind-body practices offer valuable tools for people with fibromyalgia to effectively manage pain and improve their quality of life.

INCLUDING RELAXATION METHODS IN EVERYDAY ACTIVITIES

For people with fibromyalgia, incorporating relaxation techniques into daily routines is crucial to managing stress and promoting overall well-being. Deep breathing exercises, like diaphragmatic breathing or belly breathing, help activate the body's relaxation response, calming the nervous system and reducing anxiety and stress levels. Progressive muscle relaxation is tensing and releasing muscle groups systematically, promoting physical relaxation and reducing muscle tension that contributes to pain.

Creating a daily relaxation ritual that incorporates these techniques—whether through structured sessions or brief moments throughout the day—helps individuals with fibromyalgia manage symptoms more effectively and improve their overall quality of life. Guided imagery is another useful technique where people visualize peaceful scenes or positive outcomes, engaging the mind in a relaxing and immersive experience.

This practice can lower cortisol levels and promote feelings of relaxation and well-being.

To sum up, integrating relaxation methods into everyday activities provides fibromyalgia sufferers with useful tools to handle stress and improve their overall well-being. Progressive muscle relaxation, deep breathing exercises, and guided imagery encourage physical relaxation, lessen anxiety, and aid in the body's natural healing processes. By integrating these methods into daily life, people can develop resilience, lessen the intensity of their symptoms, and become better able to handle chronic pain and exhaustion.

DEVELOPING WELL-BEING ROUTINES FOR THE LONG TERM

For people with fibromyalgia, developing healthy habits is essential to long-term well-being and symptom management. A balanced diet high in fruits, vegetables, lean proteins, and whole grains supplies vital nutrients for the immune system and energy production, and regular, capacity-based physical activity enhances cardiovascular health, muscle strength, and flexibility while easing the pain and exhaustion that come with fibromyalgia.

A consistent sleep schedule, a well-optimized sleep environment (low light and noise levels, comfortable temperature regulation, etc.), and stress management (mindfulness, relaxation, and social support) all contribute to emotional well-being and resilience in the face of chronic illness. Prioritizing adequate sleep is also crucial because restorative sleep supports immune function, cognitive function, and overall physical recovery.

Developing healthy habits helps people with fibromyalgia manage their symptoms over the long term and improve their quality of life. By emphasizing nutrition, exercise, good sleep hygiene, stress reduction, and social support, people can lessen the effects of fibromyalgia on daily activities and improve their overall quality of life.

CHAPTER NINE

MANAGING SOCIAL EVENTS WHILE FOLLOWING A DIET

It can be difficult for people with dietary restrictions to navigate social situations, particularly for those who are also managing fibromyalgia. It is crucial to communicate your dietary needs assertively and clearly while being mindful of social settings. One proactive way to manage social situations is to plan by researching the menu if you are going out to eat or notifying hosts in advance about your dietary restrictions if you are attending social gatherings. This way, you will not only avoid awkward situations but also guarantee that your dietary needs are respected.

Putting your attention on foods that help control your fibromyalgia symptoms—like anti-inflammatory foods or foods high in vitamins and minerals—will also help you stay positive and enjoy social interactions without feeling deprived.

Moreover, informing your close friends and family about your dietary needs will help them understand and support you, which will make social events more inclusive and enjoyable for everyone.

Finally, remember that navigating social situations with dietary restrictions is about advocating for your health while still fully participating in social life. Don't be afraid to bring a dish that suits your dietary needs to potlucks or parties. This will not only ensure you have something safe to eat but will also introduce others to delicious and healthy alternatives they might enjoy.

ADVICE FOR FIBROMYALGIA PATIENTS WHEN DINING OUT

For fibromyalgia patients, eating out can be both enjoyable and challenging when it comes to managing their diet. To make eating out less stressful, look for restaurants that is known for their ability to accommodate special dietary needs or that offer healthier options. A lot of restaurants these days will even customize meals based on dietary restrictions, so don't be afraid to ask about ingredient substitutions or preparation techniques that work for you.

If the portion sizes are large, consider splitting a dish with a dining partner or ordering a take-out container ahead of time to avoid overindulging.

When ordering, choose dishes that are grilled, baked, or steamed rather than fried or heavily sauced, as these cooking methods are generally healthier and easier for digestion. It's also helpful to ask for dressings and sauces on the side so you can control how much you consume.

Last but not least, ask the server or chef directly if you have any questions about the menu or ingredients; they can often offer helpful hints about how dishes are made and appropriate substitutes. Being proactive and knowledgeable can make eating out enjoyable and help you achieve your fibromyalgia management objectives.

SUPPORT FROM FRIENDS AND FAMILY FOR DIETARY ADJUSTMENTS

When it comes to managing your fibromyalgia symptoms through dietary changes, the support of friends and family is invaluable. It's critical to be transparent with them about your health objectives and dietary requirements. Educating them about fibromyalgia and how specific foods can affect symptoms can help to build understanding and promote supportive behaviors.

Involve guests in meal planning and preparation when you're hosting so that there are options that suit your dietary requirements. Sharing meals that are customized to your needs can strengthen bonds and make mealtimes enjoyable for everyone. Inspire family and friends to join you in discovering new recipes and healthy eating habits.

Remember, family and friends who are supportive can play a significant role in your overall well-being and success in managing your dietary restrictions for fibromyalgia. Having a support system that both understands and respects your dietary choices can also help alleviate any feelings of isolation or frustration that may arise from dietary restrictions.

INCLUDING DIET IN EVERYDAY ACTIVITIES

Starting with creating a meal plan that includes balanced meals with plenty of fruits, vegetables, lean proteins, and whole grains, not only ensures you're getting essential nutrients but also reduces the temptation to make unhealthy food choices out of convenience.

Including a fibromyalgia-friendly diet in daily life activities require planning and preparation but can significantly improve overall well-being.

Incorporating snacks that support stable blood sugar levels, like nuts, seeds, and yogurt, can also help maintain energy throughout the day. Meal prep can be a lifesaver when managing fibromyalgia symptoms, as it minimizes the effort needed to prepare meals on busy days. Invest in storage containers and portion out meals ahead of time so they're ready to grab and go when needed.

When you're organizing your schedule, think about how your diet can help your overall health and energy levels. Drink lots of water and herbal teas to stay hydrated. Try to work in some light exercise, like yoga or walking, to balance your diet. With a few small, sustainable adjustments to your daily routine, you can easily incorporate a fibromyalgia-friendly diet into your life and reap the benefits.

HANDLING THE EMOTIONAL SIDE OF NUTRITIONAL ADJUSTMENTS

Handling the emotional side effects of dietary modifications for managing fibromyalgia entails identifying and resolving any frustration, limitation, or sadness that may surface. It's normal to feel overwhelmed when adjusting to a new eating pattern, particularly if it means giving up favorite foods or overcoming social obstacles. Give yourself space to mourn these losses while concentrating on the gains that can enhance your quality of life and health.

Joining support groups or online communities for people with fibromyalgia can also help you connect with others who understand the challenges you're facing. Seeking guidance from healthcare professionals, such as dietitians or therapists, can provide invaluable guidance and emotional support during this transition. They can help you develop coping strategies, set realistic goals, and find alternatives to favorite foods that align with your dietary needs.

Engage in joyful and relaxing activities, such as reading, going outside, or taking up creative hobbies. Keep in mind that adapting to dietary changes is a journey, and it's important to be kind to yourself throughout the process. With time and support, you can adapt to your new dietary regimen and thrive despite any emotional challenges that may arise. Practice self-care techniques, such as mindfulness meditation or journaling, to manage stress and promote emotional well-being.

CHAPTER TEN

MATERIALS AND ASSISTANCE

FURTHER READING AND RESOURCES FOR PEOPLE WITH FIBROMYALGIA

There are a lot of resources available to assist you in managing your fibromyalgia through diet, but navigating a diagnosis can be confusing. Start with reliable sources, such as medical websites, journals, and books that focus on fibromyalgia and nutrition. These resources can offer you insights into dietary approaches that can help with symptoms like fatigue and chronic pain. Look for evidence-based information that emphasizes balanced nutrition, including lists of essential nutrients and food groups that are beneficial for managing fibromyalgia.

Look into cookbooks that are specific to fibromyalgia diets because they provide useful recipes and meal plans that assist with managing symptoms. These cookbooks typically contain simple-to-make recipes that are low in processed sugars and refined carbohydrates, emphasizing whole foods that are high in antioxidants and anti-inflammatory qualities. Moreover, fibromyalgia-related websites and forums frequently have community-recommended resources and individual success stories that offer helpful advice and inspiration for those starting the process of making dietary adjustments.

Prioritize peer-reviewed publications and clinical studies that investigate how particular diets affect fibromyalgia symptoms when conducting research. These studies can provide scientific validation as well as useful strategies for putting into practice dietary changes that are in line with your health objectives.

By remaining knowledgeable and utilizing a range of resources, you can empower yourself with knowledge and make well-informed decisions about your dietary choices to effectively manage fibromyalgia.

Joining local or online support groups allows you to share experiences, trade recipes, and learn from others who have successfully adapted their diets to alleviate symptoms. These communities often foster a sense of belonging and understanding, helping you navigates the complexities of dietary changes with compassion and solidarity. Making connections with people who understand the challenges of living with fibromyalgia can provide invaluable emotional support and practical advice on dietary management.

You can ask questions, look for recommendations for fibromyalgia-friendly recipes, and learn about new research on nutrition and its effect on fibromyalgia symptoms by participating in the many online forums and social media groups devoted to fibromyalgia. These communities also provide peer support networks, discussions on diet modifications, and expert advice from healthcare professionals specializing in chronic pain management.

Active participation in support groups and online communities can help you create a supportive network that empowers you to make informed decisions and maintain a positive outlook on your journey toward better health. Support groups also offer opportunities to participate in virtual events like webinars and live chats with nutritionists and dietitians who specialize in fibromyalgia. These sessions can offer personalized guidance on crafting meal plans tailored to your specific needs and preferences, ensuring that your dietary adjustments support overall health and symptom relief.

LOCATING MEDICAL EXPERTS WITH DIETARY MANAGEMENT EXPERIENCE

To create a customized nutrition plan that fits your specific needs, work with healthcare professionals who specialize in dietary management and fibromyalgia. Rheumatologists, nutritionists, and dietitians are examples of healthcare professionals who have treated patients with chronic pain conditions like fibromyalgia and can provide knowledgeable advice on dietary strategies that support overall well-being and symptom management.

When selecting a healthcare provider, give preference to those who treat fibromyalgia holistically, with nutrition playing a major role in their care plans. You can get referrals from your primary care physician, ask around for recommendations from fibromyalgia-focused online forums and local support groups, and look for providers who will listen to your concerns carefully, work with you to create realistic dietary goals, and offer ongoing support as you follow through with and modify your nutrition plan.

With the help of telemedicine platforms, you can arrange virtual consultations with specialists from anywhere in the world, providing easy access to professional advice from the comfort of your home. During these virtual consultations, you can discuss your dietary challenges, receive personalized recommendations, and track your progress with the support of a knowledgeable healthcare team committed to improving your quality of life. Technology can also be a major factor in connecting you with healthcare professionals experienced in fibromyalgia dietary management.

USING TECHNOLOGY TO TRACK AND PLAN MEALS

Using technology to help with meal planning can make managing dietary adjustments for fibromyalgia easier. Meal planning apps with features like customizable recipes, shopping lists of ingredients, and tools for nutritional analysis can help create balanced meals based on your needs and preferences more easily, which will make it easier to keep up a consistent eating schedule. You can also use food tracking apps to keep an eye on your daily intake, identify triggers for your symptoms, and spot patterns that could be affecting your fibromyalgia symptoms. Using technology to assist with meal planning and tracking can help you make educated food choices, stay on top of your diet, and modify recipes to meet your nutritional objectives and personal preferences.

To effectively navigate challenges, it is important to address common concerns and questions regarding dietary management for fibromyalgia. To start, make a list of frequently asked questions based on your specific dietary needs. You can also get accurate information by consulting reputable sources, such as healthcare providers or reputable health websites. Common concerns include managing flare-ups through diet, identifying trigger foods, modifying recipes to accommodate dietary restrictions, and ensuring nutritional adequacy while avoiding exacerbation of symptoms. To address these concerns, try experimenting with different foods, keeping an eye on symptom responses, and making dietary adjustments under professional guidance to optimize symptom management and overall well-being.

www.ingramcontent.com/pod-product-compliance
Lightning Source LLC
Chambersburg PA
CBHW061254250726
48653CB00002B/657